GUIDES ON HOW TO BUILD YOUR SELF-ESTEEM
Illustrative Guides On How To Boost Your Self-Esteem

Kossy Eze

Table Of Content

Chapter 1

WHAT IS SELF-ESTEEM

Strong self-esteem is the foundation upon which a fulfilling and successful life is built. It impacts mental and physical health, relationships, career, and overall well-being. Cultivating and maintaining healthy self-esteem is an
investment in one's present and future happiness.

Self-esteem is what we think of ourselves. When it's positive, we have confidence and self-respect. We're content with ourselves and our abilities, who we are, and our competence. Self-esteem is relatively stable and enduring, though it can fluctuate. Healthy self-esteem makes us resilient and hopeful about life. Self-esteem affects not only what we think, but also how we feel and behave. It has significant ramifications for our happiness and enjoyment of life. It considerably affects events in our lives, including our relationships, our work and goals, and how we care for ourselves. Although difficult events, such as breakups, illness, or loss of income, may in the short term moderate our self-esteem, we soon rebound to think positively about ourselves and our future. Even when we fail, it doesn't diminish our self-esteem. People with healthy self-esteem credit themselves when things go right, and when they don't, they consider external causes and also honestly evaluate their mistakes and shortcomings. Then they improve upon them. Self Esteem is the satisfaction or dissatisfaction with oneself" (James – 1980). Self-esteem is the judgment or opinion we hold about ourselves. It's the extent to which we perceive ourselves to be worthwhile and capable human beings."

(Coopersmith, 1967)

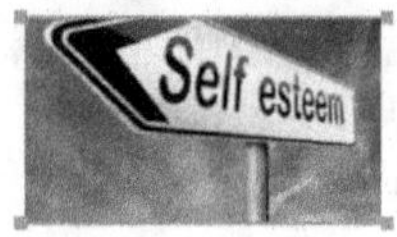

FACTORS INFLUENCING SELF ESTEEM

Self-esteem or self-image of adolescents is based on six domains as shown in Figure 2.

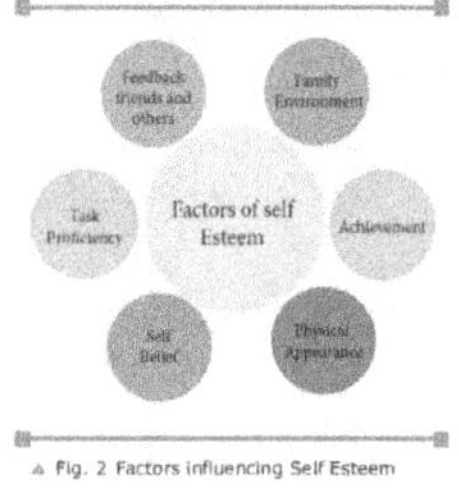

△ Fig. 2 Factors influencing Self Esteem

FAMILY ENVIRONMENT

Family is the first school for an individual. A child's life is mainly influenced by the family environment; it is the primary source of social development. Each family is different from the other, as it is composed of different members. Each varies in its social and economic conditions with different background

ACHIEVEMENT

Academic achievement and achievement of one's goals related to their hobbies play a crucial role in forming a positive, healthy view of the self.

PHYSICAL APPEARANCE

Physical characteristics such as hair, figure height wWeskinand skin color may also influence the self-esteem of an individual

SELF BELIEF

A person who has high confidence levels may learn things quickly, and rust that they can complete tasks to a good standard and this subsequently may boost their self-esteem

TASK PROFICIENCY

This includes the skills required for performing tasks and the ability to complete the task. Task proficiency influences the personality of an individual

FEEDBACK FROM FRIENDS

Positive and negative messages and feedback from friends and others may boost or break an individual's self-esteem.

Chapter 2

HEALTHY Vs IMPAIRED SELF ESTEEM

I prefer to use the terms healthy and impaired self-esteem, rather than high and low because narcissists and conceited individuals who appear to have high self-esteem don't. Theirs are inflated, compensate for shame and insecurity, and are often unrelated to reality. Boasting is an example because it indicates that the person is dependent on others' opinions of them and reveals impaired rather than healthy self-esteem. Thus, healthy self-esteem requires that we're able to honestly and realistically assess our strengths and weaknesses. We're not too concerned about others' opinions of us. When we accept our flaws without judgment, our self-acceptance goes beyond self-esteem.

IMPAIRED SELF-ESTEEM

Impaired self-esteem negatively impacts our ability to manage adversity and life's disappointments. All of our relationships are affected, including our relationship with ourselves. When our self-esteem is impaired, we feel insecure, compare ourselves to others, and doubt and criticize ourselves. We neither recognize our worth, nor honor and express our needs and wants. Instead, we may self-sacrifice, defer to others, or try to control them and/or their feelings toward us to feel better about ourselves. For example, we might please people, manipulate, or devalue them, provoke jealousy, or restrict their association with others. Consciously or unconsciously, we devalue ourselves, including our positive skills and attributes, making us hyper-sensitive to criticism. We may also be afraid to try new things because we might fail.

CAUSES OF IMPAIRED SELF-ESTEEM

Growing up in a dysfunctional family can lead to codependency as an adult. It also weakens your self-esteem. Often you don't have a voice. Your opinions and desires aren't taken seriously. Parents usually have low self-esteem and are unhappy with each other. They neither have nor model good relationship skills, including cooperation, healthy boundaries, assertiveness, and conflict resolution. They may be abusive, controlling, interfering, manipulative, indifferent, inconsistent, or just preoccupied. Directly or indirectly, they may shame their children's feelings and personal traits, feelings, and needs. It's not safe to be, to trust, and to express themselves.

Children feel insecure, anxious, and/or angry. As a result, they feel emotionally abandoned and conclude that they are at fault, and not good enough to be acceptable to both parents. (They might still believe that they're loved.) Eventually, they don't like themselves and feel inferior or inadequate. They grow up codependent with low self-esteem and learn to hide their feelings, walk on eggshells, withdraw, and try to please or become aggressive. This reflects how toxic shame becomes internalized.

Self Esteem can be classified as HIGH SELF-ESTEEM and LOW SELF_ESTEEM

SELF ESTEEM

HIGH SELF-ESTEEM	LOW SELF_ESTEEM
1. Worthy of living	1. Poor risk taker
2. Self confident	2. Afraid of competitions or challenges
3. Accept themselves unconditionally	3. Non-Assertive
4. Seek continuous self-improvement	4. Lack initiative
5. Have peace with in themselves	5. Shyness
6. Enjoy good interpersonal relationship	6. Lack self-acceptance
7. Tolerate frustrations well	7. Blame others for their short comings
8. Assertive	8. Low aspiration
9. Willing to take calculated risks	9. Indifferent to needs of others
10. Self directed	10. Indecisive

CHAPTER 3

GUIDES ON HOW TO BUILD SELF-ESTEEM

VALUE YOURSELF INTERNALLY AND EXTERNALLY

To do that, you must stop comparing yourself to others. When you compare yourself to others, the first thing you will notice is their superiority and your shortcomings, and if you do it consistently, then each time you will find more reasons to hate your life. By loving yourself, I do not mean becoming selfish or egoistic, but rather accepting who you are. It becomes a habit over time, and you are unable to judge yourself or your activities and their effects objectively as a result. This behavior causes you to fully lose confidence in yourself and your ability to succeed, as you cease believing in yourself. Let's imagine you were hired by a corporation, and in your department, your coworkers had already accumulated an apartment, a car, and trips abroad. What sort of ideas might you have after viewing such a scenario? Although you may be a recent graduate and therefore have more energy, time, or talent than anyone else in the company, you unconsciously started looking at others as better than you, and that could have serious damage to your self-esteem. If you don't accept yourself for who you are, then don't expect others to either. As a result, you may start to feel like a loser and that you haven't accomplished anything in your life, despite your advantages. To achieve this for yourself, you must stop comparing yourself to others. The only person to whom you can compare yourself is your previous self, and the only outcome to which you can compare yourself is your previous result. Valuing yourself internally and externally means recognizing your worth and acknowledging your positive qualities. This can greatly contribute to boosting self-esteem because when you value yourself internally, you develop a positive self-image and a stronger sense of self-worth. This allows you to have a more realistic and balanced view of yourself, focusing on your strengths rather than solely on your perceived weaknesses.

When you value yourself externally, you seek validation and acceptance from others based on your true worth.

This means surrounding yourself with people who appreciate and support you, and engaging in activities or pursuing goals that align with your values and satisfy you. By valuing yourself both internally and externally, you are reinforcing the belief that you deserve respect and positive treatment from others, which further enhances your self-esteem.

Valuing yourself both internally and externally can be a great way to boost your self-esteem. Here are some of the ways it can help:

INTERNAL VALIDATION: When you value yourself internally, you develop a strong sense of self-worth that isn't dependent on other people's opinions. This means recognizing and appreciating your strengths, abilities, and accomplishments. This internal validation helps build a positive self-image and increases self-esteem.

SETTING HEALTHY BOUNDARIES: Valuing yourself both internally and externally helps you set healthy boundaries in relationships and interactions. It allows you to assert yourself, communicate your needs, and prevent others from taking advantage of you. This builds self-respect and enhances self-esteem.

Developing and maintaining healthy boundaries is crucial for building self-esteem. Identify your values and priorities and Take the time to reflect on what is important to you and what you will and won't tolerate in your life. Knowing your values and priorities will help you set boundaries aligned with who you are and what you believe in. Learn to say no: Practice saying no without feeling guilty or needing to provide elaborate explanations. It's okay to decline requests or activities that don't align with your values or personal needs. Saying no assertively and without guilt helps establish boundaries and protects your time and energy. Communicate your boundaries and Clearly express your boundaries to others respectfully and communicate your needs, expectations, and limits explicitly so that others understand where you stand. It's important to communicate your boundaries continuously, as people may forget or inadvertently cross them. Be assertive in communication, Develop assertive communication skills to convey your boundaries effectively. Be clear, direct, and confident in expressing your thoughts, opinions, and boundaries. Avoid being aggressive or passive, as these communication styles can lead to misunderstandings and difficulties in maintaining healthy boundaries. Establish consequences for boundary violations. If someone constantly crosses or disrespects your boundaries, it's important to establish consequences for their actions. Communicate and enforce these consequences to demonstrate that your boundaries are non-negotiable. Consistency is key in unfolding boundaries and maintaining self-esteem.

Remember, setting and maintaining boundaries takes practice and assertiveness. Be patient with yourself and keep reinforcing your boundaries to protect your self-esteem and overall well-being.

EMBRACING SELF-ACCEPTANCE: When you value yourself internally, you cultivate self-acceptance and self-compassion. You learn to embrace your flaws, imperfections, and vulnerabilities, realizing that they don't determine your worth. Acceptance and compassion contribute to increased self-esteem.

CELEBRATING ACHIEVEMENTS: By valuing yourself externally, you acknowledge and celebrate your achievements and milestones. You take pride in your accomplishments, giving yourself credit for your hard work and dedication. Recognizing your successes helps boost self-esteem by reinforcing a positive self-image

SURROUNDING YOURSELF WITH POSITIVITY: Valuing yourself internally and externally encourages you to prioritize your well-being by surrounding yourself with positive influences and environments. This means seeking out supportive relationships, engaging in activities that bring you joy and fulfillment, and avoiding toxic situations. Being in a positive environment nurtures self-esteem and self-confidence.

BUILDING RESILIENCE: Valuing yourself both internally and externally contributes to building resilience. When you have a solid foundation of self-worth, you are better equipped to handle challenges, setbacks, and criticism. You are more likely to bounce back from failures, maintain a positive outlook, and continue to believe in yourself.

Building resilience is a crucial component of building self-esteem because it helps individuals bounce back from setbacks and challenges.

Embrace failure as a learning opportunity and Shift your perspective on failure from something negative to an opportunity for growth. View setbacks as valuable lessons and adjust your approach accordingly. Remember that failure is a natural part of life and it does not define your worth. Cultivate a supportive network. Surround yourself with positive and supportive people who uplift and encourage you. Seek out friends, family, or mentors who believe in you and provide support during challenging times.

Develop problem-solving skills to Enhance your ability to problem-solve by breaking problems down into smaller, more manageable parts. Seek creative solutions and make a plan of action. The more confident you are in your ability to solve problems, the more resilient you become.

Practice gratitude and Cultivating a mindset of gratitude can help you focus on the positive aspects of your life and build resilience. Regularly reflect on and appreciate the things you are thankful for. This can help shift your perspective during difficult times.

Practice stress management techniques, Different techniques such as deep breathing exercises, meditation, or engaging in activities that help you relax can help manage stress and enhance resilience. These techniques can help you stay grounded and provide a sense of inner peace. By developing resilience, you can navigate life's challenges with confidence, which in turn builds self-esteem. Remember that building resilience is an ongoing process that takes time and practice.

In conclusion, valuing yourself internally and externally can be a great way to boost your self-esteem. By recognizing your worth and abilities, setting healthy boundaries, practicing self-acceptance, celebrating achievements surrounding yourself with positivity, and building resilience, you can greatly enhance your self-esteem and overall well-being.

CHAPTER 4

STOP BERATING YOURSELF FOR SMALL MISTAKES

Permit mistakes to happen to you. This idea of achieving perfection in everything is absurd. Stop being hard on yourself for making a few minor mistakes. Everyone would like to be the best at everything they do, but that isn't possible. Instead, focus on developing your strengths. If you make a lot of mistakes throughout your life, don't get discouraged; that's how we learn.

On the other hand, putting an end to self-criticism is crucial for increasing self-esteem since it enables you to have compassion for yourself. Self-criticism frequently entails negative self-talk that emphasizes your mistakes or flaws, which can over time foster a negative outlook and lower your self-esteem. Stopping your self-criticism allows you to develop self-compassion and kindness.

You can adopt a more realistic and fair attitude rather than criticize yourself for your perceived flaws. Recognize that learning and growing include making mistakes, which is a normal and important component of both. You can cultivate a more positive self-image and boost your self-esteem by changing your perspective to place more emphasis on self-improvement than self-judgment. It is essential to embrace who you are and recognize your abilities and accomplishments if you want to develop a stronger sense of self-worth.

Instead of berating yourself for your perceived shortcomings, you can adopt a more realistic and balanced perspective. Recognize that making mistakes is a natural and necessary part of growth and learning. By shifting your mindset to focus on self-improvement rather than self-judgment, you can foster a more positive self-image and nurture your self-esteem. Embracing self-acceptance and acknowledging your strengths and achievements are crucial steps toward building healthier self-esteem. Building self-esteem requires being kind and forgiving towards yourself. One way to do this is by stopping the habit of berating yourself for small mistakes. Accept imperfections and Recognize that nobody is perfect, and striving for perfection is unrealistic and exhausting. Embrace your imperfections as unique qualities that make you who you are.

Focus on achievements and Acknowledge and celebrate your accomplishments, both big and small. Shift your focus toward your strengths and the things you are proud of, rather than dwelling on the mistakes or shortcomings.

Set realistic expectations and do well to avoid setting unrealistic expectations for yourself. Be mindful of what is genuinely achievable within the realm of your abilities and circumstances. Setting realistic goals can help you avoid unnecessary disappointment and self-criticism.

QUIT GRIPING ABOUT YOUR LIFE

Some people gripe about everything in life, including their families, neighborhoods, bad friends, and an unending list of other grievances. The saying goes, "What you can achieve without complaining is pity from others." I don't believe it's something you want but keep in mind that if people feel sorry for you, they will perceive you as a loser.

Complaining often comes from a sense of entitlement or not being thankful for what you have. When you stop complaining, you can start to be grateful for the good things in your life. This can make you feel content and improve your overall well-being. The more you practice gratitude and positivity, the better your self-esteem will be.

Not complaining can help you feel more empowered and take ownership of your life. Complaining can make you feel like a victim like you don't have any control over your happiness. But if you stop complaining, you can start to recognize that you have the power to change your circumstances and make your life better. This can help you feel more confident and create a more fulfilling life.

All in all, if you stop complaining about your life, you can create a more positive mindset, develop problem-solving skills, foster gratitude and self-empowerment, and promote personal growth. All of these things can help you build your self-esteem and create a more confident sense of self.

TAKE UP A HOBBY OR OTHER ACTIVITIES YOU ENJOY DOING

If you wake up every morning to do something you detest for the entire day, you can never have great self-esteem. Find a better career or strive to appreciate what you are doing. Although it can be a little uncomfortable, switching professions will, in some ways, be beneficial. Engaging in activities that you find enjoyable can be a great way to increase self-esteem in a variety of ways. Doing something that you excel at can give you a sense of accomplishment and satisfaction, which can help reinforce your capabilities and talents. Additionally, when you pursue activities that you enjoy, you often interact with others who share your interests or appreciate your skills, which can provide you with positive feedback and recognition, validating your abilities and giving you a sense of importance. Furthermore, engaging in activities that you enjoy allows you to express yourself freely, unleashing your creativity and individuality, which can foster a sense of authenticity and confidence in your abilities. Additionally, pursuing activities that you enjoy can result in personal growth and development as you invest time and effort into something you love and witness your growth and development. Finally, engaging in activities that you enjoy leads to greater fulfillment and happiness, creating a positive perception of yourself and your abilities, which can improve self-esteem. In conclusion, doing something you enjoy can provide a sense of accomplishment, positive feedback, self-expression, personal growth, and enjoyable experiences, all of which can help boost self-esteem.

EMBRACE YOUR BODY, MIND AND SOUL

The only way to embrace who you are is to respect your body, mind, and soul. Living a healthy lifestyle is essential to respect your body. Get rid of alcohol, cigarettes, and anything else that is bad for your health. It makes no difference what it is. Spend at least three hours in the gym each week. Not only will you feel amazing when your muscles begin to develop, but you'll also feel as though your muscles are being used to their full potential, which will boost your confidence and sense of self-worth. When it comes to feeding your head and your spirit, read literature.

Focusing on your strengths: By emphasizing your talents and achievements, you can develop a positive self-image and appreciate your unique qualities.

Acknowledging external validation: Receiving compliments, praise, and recognition from others can affirm your worthiness and capabilities, and remind you that others see and appreciate your value.

Practicing self-compassion: Treating yourself with kindness, care, and understanding helps to nurture a healthier perspective of yourself and boost self-esteem.

Prioritizing self-care: Taking care of all aspects of your well-being demonstrates self-respect and enhances your overall sense of self-worth.

Setting and achieving goals: Pursuing and achieving meaningful goals validates your abilities and capabilities, leading to a stronger sense of self-esteem.

Establishing healthy boundaries: Asserting your needs, desires, and limits communicates your self-worth and demands the respect you deserve. This assertiveness reinforces your belief in your value.

In conclusion, Embracing Your Body, Mind, And Soul is a powerful way to increase your self-esteem. It involves recognizing and appreciating your worth, practicing self-compassion, prioritizing self-care, setting and achieving goals, establishing g het, abound and. Through these practices, you can cultivate a stronger sense of self-esteem

Building self-esteem involves taking care of not only our physical appearance but also our mental and emotional well-being. Embracing our mind and soul is essential in the journey of building self-esteem.

Cultivate self-awareness. Reflect on your thoughts, feelings, and behaviors. Understand your strengths and areas for growth. This self-awareness can help you build confidence and make positive changes.

Focus on personal growth and set aside time for self-reflection, personal development, and learning. Investing in your growth and acquiring new skills can boost your self-esteem.

POSITIVE SELF TALK

Pat Yourself at the back When you accomplish something, don't give the credit to luck, give it to yourself. Don't think that if you succeeded in something it was because of luck. Sure, there may be some external factors, but it was you who put in the hard work and effort. If you still don't believe it, write down your accomplishments, but don't go overboard and start having an ego issue.

Identify negative thoughts, Start by becoming aware of the negative thoughts or self-talk that frequently crops up in your mind. Pay attention to the specific phrases or statements that bring you down, such as "I'm not good enough," "I always mess up," or "I'll never succeed."

Question the validity: Once you catch these negative thoughts, objectively question their validity. Ask yourself if there is any concrete evidence supporting these thoughts. Often, you'll find that they are based on assumptions, insecurities, or past experiences that may not accurately reflect your current reality.

Find alternative perspectives. Now, actively seek alternative perspectives or counterarguments to challenge your

negative thoughts. For example, if you think, "I'm not
good enough," remind yourself of past successes or
achievements that contradict this belief. Look for evidence
that emphasizes your strengths, talents, or positive
qualities.

Replace with positive affirmations. Once you've identified
alternative perspectives, replace the negative thoughts with
positive affirmations. Develop a list of positive statements
about yourself that counter the negative self-talk. Repeat
these affirmations regularly to reinforce positive
self-beliefs.

PRACTICE SELF COMPASSION AND ACCEPTANCE

Recognize that no one is perfect, including yourself.
Embrace self-compassion and self-acceptance by
acknowledging that making mistakes is a natural part of
growth. Treat yourself with kindness and understanding.
Recognize that everyone has flaws and makes mistakes
and that it's a normal part of being human. Offer yourself
the same care and support you would extend to a friend in
a similar situation.

Start with self-awareness. Notice when you are being self-critical or engaging in negative self-talk. Pay attention to the thoughts and words you use while evaluating yourself. Replace self-criticism with self-compassion: When you catch yourself being self-critical, consciously shift your mindset towards self-compassion. Treat yourself with kindness, empathy, and understanding.

Cultivate mindfulness, Practice being present in the moment without judgment. This can help you become aware of your emotions and thoughts while detached from them, allowing you to respond with compassion instead of self-criticism.

Challenge negative beliefs: Identify and question negative beliefs or limiting self-perceptions. Explore where they come from and consider alternative, more balanced perspectives that are kinder to yourself.

Practice self-acceptance. Embrace yourself as you are, along with your strengths, weaknesses, and imperfections. Recognize that everyone has flaws and that they do not define your worth or value as a person.

AVOID COMPARISON

Comparing yourself to others can weaken self-esteem. Remember that everyone has unique strengths and weaknesses, and it's unproductive to measure your worth based on someone else's success or appearance. Instead, focus on your journey and progress.

One way to boost your self-esteem is to avoid comparing yourself to others. Comparison often leads to negative thoughts and feelings about ourselves, as we tend to focus on our perceived shortcomings or deficiencies compared to others. Instead, recognize and embrace your unique qualities, strengths, and accomplishments. Appreciate your progress and growth, and celebrate your successes no matter how small they may seem. Additionally, surrounding yourself with positive and supportive people who uplift and encourage you can also contribute to boosting your self-esteem. Remember to practice self-care, engage in activities that you enjoy, and set realistic and achievable goals for yourself. Finally, treat yourself with kindness, compassion, and love, and practice positive self-talk to build a more positive self-perception. Embrace your uniqueness. Instead of comparing yourself to others, appreciate your individuality. Recognize that everyone has different strengths, talents, and qualities that make them special. Focus on celebrating and showcasing what makes you unique.

Prioritize self-care, Take care of yourself both mentally and physically. Engage in activities that make you feel good, such as exercising regularly, eating nourishing foods, getting enough sleep, and practicing relaxation techniques like meditation or yoga. When you prioritize self-care, you'll naturally feel more confident and positive about yourself.

Dress for yourself and Wear clothes that make you feel comfortable, and confident, and express your style. Don't base your fashion choices solely on the latest trends or what others are wearing. Choose outfits that make you feel good about yourself and reflect your personality. Practice good hygiene. Taking care of your hygiene can have a positive impact on your self-esteem. Make it a habit to maintain good oral hygiene, shower regularly, groom yourself, and dress neatly. Feeling clean and fresh can help boost your self-confidence.

Accept compliments gracefully When someone compliments you, accept it graciously and believe in their words. Avoid dismissing or downplaying compliments as this undermines your self-esteem. Instead, say thank you and internalize the positive feedback. Focus on your strengths and Shift your focus from your perceived flaws to your strengths and accomplishments. Acknowledge and appreciate your unique talents, skills, and abilities. Write them down and remind yourself of your positive attributes regularly. Set achievable and realistic goals for yourself can help build confidence and self-esteem. Break them down into smaller, manageable steps and celebrate each milestone you achieve. This will reinforce a sense of accomplishment and boost your self-confidence.

TAKE CARE OF YOUR PHYSICAL APPEARANCE

Taking care of your physical appearance can contribute to feeling more confident. Dress in a way that makes you feel good about yourself and practice good hygiene.
Taking care of your physical appearance can positively impact your self-esteem.
Practice good grooming, Pay attention to your presence, such as bathing regularly, brushing your teeth, and maintaining clean and neat hair.

Dress in a way that makes you feel confident: Wear clothes that make you feel comfortable and express your purse. Dressing to impress yourself can boost your self-esteem.

Take care of your body, Engage in regular physical activity that you enjoy, such as going for walks, doing yoga, or participating in sports. Exercise releases endorphins, which can improve your mood and self-confidence.

Eat a balanced diet. Nourishing your body with healthy and nutritious food can improve your overall well-being and enhance your self-esteem.

Get enough sleep. Prioritize getting adequate sleep to ensure you wake up feeling refreshed and rejuvenated. Lack of sleep can negatively impact your self-confidence and mood.

Remember, while taking care of your physical appearance is important, self-esteem is not solely based on external factors. It's also essential to focus on building a strong internal foundation.

SEEK PROFESSIONAL HELP IF NECESSARY

If low self-esteem is significantly affecting your daily life, consider seeking support from a therapist or counselor.

They can help you work through underlying issues and provide guidance on building self-esteem.

Seeking professional help can be enormously beneficial in building self-esteem. Professionals, such as therapists or counselors trained in mental health, have the knowledge and experience to support individuals in understanding and improving their self-esteem.

Professionals can help individuals assess their current level of self-esteem. Through discussions and evaluations, they can identify underlying factors that may be contributing to low self-esteem or hindering its development. This assessment is crucial as it sets the foundation for targeting specific areas of improvement.

Individualized strategies. Professionals can tailor strategies and techniques based on each individual's unique needs and challenges. They can offer evidence-based interventions that have been proven effective in boosting self-esteem. These strategies might include cognitive-behavioral therapy (CBT), positive affirmations, visualization exercises, or guided self-reflection.

Identifying core beliefs, Often, low self-esteem is rooted in negative core beliefs that individuals hold about themselves. Professionals can help individuals uncover these deep-seated beliefs and challenge their accuracy and validity. By replacing negative beliefs with more positive and empowering ones, individuals can cultivate healthier self-perceptions.

Emotional support: Professionals provide a safe and non-judgmental space for individuals to express their emotions and concerns. Through active listening and empathetic understanding, they can help individuals explore their feelings about themselves and the factors influencing their self-esteem. This emotional support can be crucial in building resilience and developing a more positive self-image.

Skill-building: Professionals can offer guidance and teach practical skills that promote self-esteem. These skills may include assertiveness training, effective communication, problem-solving, stress management, and self-care techniques. By acquiring these skills, individuals become better equipped to navigate challenges and setbacks, ultimately strengthening their self-esteem.

Long-term support and accountability: Building self-esteem is not a quick fix; it requires consistent effort and practice. Professionals can provide ongoing support and accountability, helping individuals stay motivated and sustaining their progress over time. Regular therapy sessions or check-ins can serve as important reminders and opportunities for continued personal growth.

Remember, seeking professional help does not imply weakness or inadequacy. It signifies a proactive and courageous step towards improving your self-esteem and overall well-being. Professionals offer expertise, guidance, and a supportive environment, helping individuals develop a healthier self-perception and lead more fulfilling lives.

Chapter 5

A Short Story Of A Young Girl With An Unwavering Self-Esteem.

"The Unwavering Confidence of Mary"

In a bustling city, there lived a woman named Mary. Her life was a testament to unwavering confidence, a quality that had shaped her journey in remarkable ways.

From a young age, Mary had an unshakable belief in herself. She saw challenges as opportunities to grow, never as obstacles. When she decided to start her own business, many doubted her abilities. But Mary's confidence in her entrepreneurial vision propelled her forward.

Mary's daily routine was a testament to her self-assured nature. Each morning, she stood before the mirror, looked herself in the eye, and repeated her mantra: "I am capable.

I am strong. I can overcome anything." This simple ritual set the tone for her day and reminded her of her worth.

Confidence wasn't about arrogance for Mary; it was about self-assurance. She treated others with respect and kindness, recognizing that everyone had their unique strengths. Mary's confident demeanor drew people to her. Her friends often sought her advice and admired her ability to remain composed in the face of adversity.

One of Mary's most significant achievements was her commitment to lifelong learning. She saw knowledge as a means to bolster her confidence further. Whether it was mastering a new skill or exploring a foreign culture, she embraced every opportunity to expand her horizons.

Mary's career soared to great heights because of her confidence. She took on leadership roles and inspired her team with her unwavering belief in their collective potential. Her charisma and ability to rally others made her a natural leader.

In her personal life, Mary's confidence also shone brightly. She navigated relationships with grace, knowing her self-worth and refusing to settle for less than she deserved. Her confidence attracted a partner who appreciated her for who she was and supported her aspirations.

As the years passed, Mary's confidence became a source of inspiration for many. People looked up to her not just for her accomplishments but for her unwavering belief in herself. She proved that confidence wasn't a fixed trait; it was a mindset that could be nurtured and developed.

Mary's life was a testament to the power of confidence. Her journey reminded us that when we believe in ourselves, embrace challenges, and treat others with respect, we can achieve remarkable things. She was living proof that confidence could be the key to unlocking a fulfilling and successful life.

Chapter 6

IMPORTANCE OF SELF-ESTEEM

Having strong self-esteem is of paramount importance for various aspects of one's Life

POSITIVE MENTAL HEALTH: Strong self-esteem is linked to better mental well-being. It reduces the risk of anxiety and depression and helps individuals cope with stress and setbacks more effectively.

Certainly, let's focus on the importance of strong self-esteem specifically on positive mental health:

Positive Mental Health: Strong self-esteem is a cornerstone of positive mental health. Here's why:

1.**Resilience to Stress:**Individuals with strong self-esteem are better equipped to handle stress. They have confidence in their abilities to manage challenges, reducing the negative impact of stress on their mental well-being.

2. **Reduced Anxiety:** High self-esteem is linked to lower levels of anxiety. When you believe in yourself, you're less likely to engage in self-doubt and excessive worry.

3. Lower Risk of Depression: People with strong self-esteem are less susceptible to depression. They tend to have a more positive outlook on life, which acts as a protective factor against depressive symptoms.

4. Emotional Regulation: Strong self-esteem contributes to better emotional regulation. It allows individuals to acknowledge and manage their emotions effectively, preventing emotional crises.

5. Positive Self-talk: Those with strong self-esteem engage in positive self-talk. They counter self-criticism with self-encouragement, fostering a more optimistic and mentally healthy mindset.

6. Enhanced Coping Skills: People with healthy self-esteem develop effective coping strategies. They are more likely to seek support when needed and adapt to adverse situations without losing their sense of self-worth.

7. Improved Relationships: Strong self-esteem positively impacts relationships, reducing conflicts and enhancing overall mental well-being. Healthy self-esteem enables individuals to set boundaries and communicate their needs, leading to more satisfying interpersonal connections.

8. Optimism and Life Satisfaction: Individuals with strong self-esteem tend to be more optimistic and experience greater life satisfaction. This positive outlook contributes to overall mental health and a sense of fulfillment.

9. Motivation and Goal Pursuit: Belief in oneself motivates individuals to pursue personal goals and aspirations. Achieving these goals fosters a sense of accomplishment and boosts mental well-being.

10. Reduction in Negative Self-image: High self-esteem helps combat negative self-image, a common factor in mental health issues. When you value yourself, you're less likely to engage in self-destructive behaviors or self-sabotage.

In summary, strong self-esteem is a powerful protector of positive mental health. It acts as a buffer against stress, anxiety, and depression, while also promoting emotional regulation, optimism, and healthy relationships. Investing in and nurturing self-esteem is a key strategy for maintaining and enhancing mental well-being.

2. HEALTHY RELATIONSHIP: It fosters healthy relationships because when you value yourself, you're more likely to choose and maintain relationships that are respectful and supportive.

Certainly, let's explore the importance of strong self-esteem in the context of healthy relationships: Healthy Relationships, Having strong self-esteem is vital for fostering and maintaining healthy relationships. Here's why it matters:

1. Setting Boundaries: Individuals with strong self-esteem are more likely to set and communicate healthy boundaries in their relationships. They understand their own needs and limits, which promotes respect and mutual understanding.

2. Respect and Equality: Healthy self-esteem encourages self-respect, and this extends to the relationships they engage in. Those with strong self-esteem are more inclined to seek and maintain relationships built on mutual respect and equality.

3. Avoiding Codependency: People with healthy self-esteem are less prone to codependent relationships where one person relies excessively on the other for emotional well-being. They have a strong sense of self-worth, reducing the need for external validation.

4. Effective Communication: Strong self-esteem often leads to better communication skills. Individuals are more assertive, able to express their thoughts and feelings clearly and listen actively to their partners.

5. Conflict Resolution: In healthy relationships, conflicts are inevitable, but strong self-esteem helps in resolving them constructively. Individuals with self-assurance are less likely to engage in destructive conflicts and more inclined to seek solutions.

6. Less Jealousy and Insecurity: People with strong self-esteem are generally less prone to jealousy and insecurity in their relationships. They trust their partners and themselves, reducing unnecessary conflicts and tensions.

7. Supportive Partnerships: Those with strong self-esteem tend to choose partners who support their personal growth and well-being. These relationships are often more nurturing and empowering.

8. Independence and Interdependence: Healthy self-esteem promotes a balance between independence and interdependence in relationships. Individuals can maintain their own identity while also being part of a supportive partnership.

9. Resilience in Breakups: Even in the face of relationship challenges or breakups, individuals with strong self-esteem tend to recover more quickly and maintain a positive self-image.

10. Role Modeling for Others: Healthy self-esteem in one partner can positively influence their significant other, promoting a mutually beneficial cycle of self-assurance and healthy relationship dynamics

In summary, strong self-esteem is a cornerstone of healthy relationships. It enables individuals to set boundaries, communicate effectively, and engage in partnerships built on respect and equality. Nurturing self-esteem not only benefits the individual but also contributes to the creation of positive and fulfilling relationships.

3. RESILIENCE: High self-esteem enhances resilience. People with strong self-esteem bounce back from failures and setbacks more easily, as they don't internalize them as reflections of their worth.

Resilience is a critical aspect of having strong self-esteem. Resilience refers to the ability to bounce back from adversity and cope with life's challenges. Strong self-esteem plays a pivotal role in fostering resilience in several ways:

1. Positive Self-Image: Individuals with strong self-esteem have a more positive self-image. This positive self-perception serves as a foundation during tough times, helping them maintain confidence and self-worth even when facing setbacks.

2. Optimism: People with healthy self-esteem tend to be more optimistic. They believe in their abilities to overcome challenges, which fuels their resilience. Optimism is a key factor in bouncing back from adversity.

3. Emotional Regulation: Strong self-esteem often goes hand-in-hand with effective emotional regulation. Resilient individuals can acknowledge their emotions without being overwhelmed by them. This allows them to think more clearly and make sound decisions in difficult situations.

4. Problem-Solving Skills: High self-esteem encourages proactive problem-solving. Resilient individuals see challenges as opportunities to learn and grow. They approach problems with a can-do attitude, seeking solutions rather than dwelling on the negative aspects.

5. Adaptability: People with strong self-esteem tend to be more adaptable. They're open to change and less resistant to it. This flexibility is a valuable asset when dealing with unexpected or adverse circumstances.

6. Support-Seeking Behavior: Resilient individuals are more likely to seek support when needed. They don't view asking for help as a sign of weakness. Strong self-esteem enables them to reach out to others for assistance or guidance during tough times.

7. Reduced Self-Blame: Those with strong self-esteem are less prone to self-blame when things go wrong. They understand that setbacks are part of life and don't internalize failures as reflections of their worth. This self-compassion is a key component of resilience.

8. Motivation to Overcome: Belief in oneself and one's abilities serves as a powerful motivator. Resilient individuals are driven to overcome challenges precisely because they have a strong sense of self-worth.

9. Coping Strategies: People with strong self-esteem tend to have a repertoire of effective coping strategies. They can draw upon these strategies to navigate difficult situations, reducing the impact of stress on their mental well-being.

10. Positive Feedback Loop: Resilience and self-esteem create a positive feedback loop. When individuals successfully overcome challenges, their self-esteem is reinforced, making them even more resilient in the face of future adversity.

In summary, strong self-esteem and resilience are closely intertwined. Strong self-esteem serves as a source of inner strength and positivity, enabling individuals to bounce back from setbacks, cope with adversity, and emerge from challenging situations even stronger than before.

4. MOTIVATION AND GOAL ACHIEVEMENT:

Believing in your abilities and self-worth motivates you to set and pursue challenging goals. Achieving these goals further boosts self-esteem in a positive cycle. Certainly, let's explore the importance of motivation and goal achievement about having strong self-esteem. Strong self-esteem plays a crucial role in motivating individuals and driving them to achieve their goals. Here's why it's so important:

1. Belief in Abilities: Individuals with strong self-esteem believe in their abilities. This belief serves as a powerful motivator, as they're more likely to pursue challenging goals with confidence.

2. Setting Ambitious Goals: People with healthy self-esteem tend to set more ambitious goals for themselves. They don't limit their aspirations due to self-doubt, which can lead to greater achievements.

3. Perseverance: When faced with obstacles or setbacks, those with strong self-esteem are more likely to persevere. They view challenges as opportunities to learn and grow, rather than reasons to give up.

4. Positive Self-talk: Self-assured individuals engage in positive self-talk, which reinforces their motivation. They encourage themselves, counter self-doubt, and stay focused on their objectives.

5. Resilience in the Face of Failure: Failure is a part of pursuing goals, but strong self-esteem helps individuals bounce back from failures. They don't see setbacks as personal shortcomings, making them more resilient in their pursuit of success.

6. Risk-Taking: Individuals with strong self-esteem are more willing to take calculated risks. They recognize that stepping out of their comfort zone can lead to personal growth and achievement.

7. Confidence in Decision-Making: Making decisions related to goals is easier for those with strong self-esteem. They trust their judgment and are less likely to second-guess themselves, leading to quicker progress.

8. Positive Feedback Loop: Achieving goals reinforces self-esteem. Successes serve as evidence of one's capabilities, boosting self-assurance and motivation to set and achieve even more challenging objectives.

9. Improved Focus: Strong self-esteem contributes to improved concentration and focus. Individuals are less distracted by self-doubt and negative thoughts, allowing them to work more efficiently towards their goals.

10. Personal Fulfillment: Achieving goals leads to a sense of personal fulfillment and satisfaction. People with strong self-esteem are more likely to experience a deep sense of accomplishment, contributing to their overall well-being.

In summary, strong self-esteem acts as a catalyst for motivation and goal achievement. It instills belief in one's abilities, encourages ambitious goal-setting, fosters resilience in the face of challenges, and creates a positive feedback loop of success. Nurturing self-esteem is a powerful way to propel oneself toward personal and professional achievements.

5. CONFIDENCE: Self-esteem is the foundation of confidence. It empowers you to express your opinions, take risks, and face challenges with a positive attitude. Let's explore the importance of confidence about having strong self-esteem. Confidence is a direct outcome of strong self-esteem, and it plays a pivotal role in various aspects of life. Here's why it's essential:

1. Assertiveness: Confident individuals are more assertive. They can express their thoughts, feelings, and needs effectively, which is crucial for healthy communication and setting boundaries in relationships.

2. Taking Initiative: Confidence empowers individuals to take the initiative. They are more likely to step forward and lead, whether it's in a team project at work or taking charge of their personal goals.

3. Effective Decision-Making: Confidence enhances decision-making. Those with strong self-esteem trust their judgment, which leads to quicker, more decisive choices.

4. Risk-Taking: Confident individuals are more willing to take calculated risks. They understand that success often requires stepping out of one's comfort zone, and they have the self-assurance to do so.

5. Public Speaking and Presentation Skills: Confidence is crucial for public speaking and effective presentations. It enables individuals to speak with authority and captivate their audience.

6. Career Advancement: In the workplace, confidence often translates to career success. Confident individuals are more likely to take on leadership roles and advocate for their professional growth.

7. Interpersonal Relationships: Confidence enhances interpersonal relationships. It can make someone more approachable, likable, and respected by others, leading to more fulfilling personal connections.

8. Positive Outlook: Confidence contributes to a positive outlook on life. Confident individuals tend to see

opportunities where others may see obstacles, leading to a
more optimistic and proactive approach to challenges.

9. Mental Well-being: Confidence is linked to better
mental health. It reduces self-doubt and anxiety, leading to
improved overall well-being.

10. Motivation: Confidence is a key motivator. Believing
in one's abilities and self-worth provides the drive to
pursue goals and overcome obstacles.

In summary, confidence, which is a direct result of strong
self-esteem, is a fundamental quality that enhances various
aspects of life. It empowers individuals to navigate
challenges, make decisions, pursue goals, build positive
relationships, and maintain overall well-being with a sense
of self-assuredness.

6. PHYSICAL HEALTH: Surprisingly, self-esteem can
influence physical health. Those with high self-esteem are
more likely to engage in healthy behaviors like exercise and
balanced nutrition. While self-esteem primarily addresses
psychological aspects, it can indirectly impact physical
health in several ways:

1. Healthy Lifestyle Choices: Individuals with strong self-esteem are more likely to make healthy lifestyle choices. They value themselves and their well-being, leading to behaviors like regular exercise, balanced nutrition, and adequate rest.

2. Stress Management: Strong self-esteem contributes to better stress management. Confident individuals are less prone to chronic stress, which can have detrimental effects on physical health.

3. Resilience to Illness: Research suggests that those with a positive self-image may experience enhanced immune function, which can help the body defend against illnesses.

4. Pain Tolerance: Some studies have shown that individuals with high self-esteem may have a higher pain tolerance, potentially making them more resilient in the face of physical discomfort or pain.

5. Recovery from Illness: People with strong self-esteem often exhibit a more positive attitude during illness, which can aid in the recovery process. A positive mindset can sometimes lead to faster healing.

6. Reduced Risky Behaviors: High self-esteem is associated with reduced engagement in risky behaviors such as substance abuse or reckless driving, which can directly impact physical health and safety.

7. Better Sleep: Confidence and self-assurance often translate into better sleep patterns. Quality sleep is essential for overall physical health and well-being.

8. Longevity: Some studies suggest that individuals with higher self-esteem may have a longer life expectancy, possibly due to healthier lifestyle choices and better overall health practices.

9. Enhanced Physical Performance: Self-assured individuals may experience enhanced physical performance, whether in sports, exercise, or daily activities, due to their belief in their abilities.

10. Reduced Psychosomatic Symptoms: Strong self-esteem can reduce psychosomatic symptoms, where psychological stressors manifest as physical symptoms. Improved mental well-being can alleviate these issues.

In summary, while self-esteem primarily addresses the psychological realm, its impact on physical health is significant. Strong self-esteem can lead to healthier lifestyle choices, better stress management, and improved physical well-being. A positive self-image and sense of self-worth contribute to a holistic approach to health that benefits both the mind and body.

7. **CAREER SUCCESS**: Confidence and self-assuredness are often keys to career advancement. People with strong self-esteem tend to perform better, take on leadership roles, and advocate for their needs in the workplace. Strong self-esteem is a powerful catalyst for achieving success in one's career. Here's why it's crucial:

1. Confidence in Abilities: Individuals with strong self-esteem have confidence in their skills and abilities. This self-assuredness enables them to take on challenges and pursue career opportunities with a belief in their capacity to excel.

2. Assertiveness: Confidence fosters assertiveness, a valuable trait in the workplace. Assertive individuals are more likely to express their ideas, take initiative, and advocate for their professional growth.

3. Effective Communication: Those with strong self-esteem tend to communicate more effectively. They can articulate their thoughts and ideas clearly, which is essential for collaboration and leadership roles.

4. Adaptability: Confidence makes individuals more adaptable in the face of change. They are open to new ideas, technologies, and work methods, which is crucial in a rapidly evolving job market.

5. Leadership: Strong self-esteem is often a hallmark of effective leaders. Confident leaders inspire their teams, make decisions with conviction, and navigate challenges with poise.

6. Networking: Self-assured individuals are often more proactive in networking. They confidently build relationships and seek out mentors, which can lead to valuable career opportunities.

7. Negotiation Skills: Confidence is beneficial in negotiation situations, such as salary discussions or contract agreements. Those with strong self-esteem are more likely to negotiate effectively for their benefit.

8. Job Satisfaction: Career success often leads to greater job satisfaction. Individuals with strong self-esteem tend to feel more fulfilled and content with their professional achievements.

9. Positive Work Environment: Confidence can contribute to a positive work environment. Confident individuals are often more collaborative, respectful, and supportive of their colleagues, creating a more harmonious workplace.

10. Continuous Learning: Confidence encourages a growth mindset. Those with strong self-esteem are more likely to embrace continuous learning and seek out opportunities for personal and professional development.

In summary, strong self-esteem is a cornerstone of career success. It empowers individuals to pursue their professional goals with confidence, navigate challenges effectively, and excel in leadership roles. Investing in and nurturing self-esteem is a key strategy for advancing one's career and achieving long-term success.

8. **LIFE SATISFACTION**: High self-esteem is correlated with greater life satisfaction. It leads to a sense of self-fulfillment and contentment. Let's explore the importance of strong self-esteem and life satisfaction. Strong self-esteem is closely linked to overall life satisfaction and well-being. Here's why it's crucial:

1. Optimism: Confidence and self-assurance often lead to greater optimism. Confident individuals tend to see opportunities and positives in various life situations, which enhances their overall satisfaction.

2. Healthy Relationships: Self-esteem contributes to healthier relationships. When individuals value themselves, they are more likely to establish and maintain positive, supportive connections with others, enhancing overall life satisfaction.

3. Goal Achievement: Confidence in one's abilities drives motivation to set and achieve goals. The fulfillment of achieving these goals can significantly boost life satisfaction.

4. Lower Anxiety and Depression: Strong self-esteem is associated with lower levels of anxiety and depression. Reduced mental health issues contribute to an improved overall sense of well-being.

5. Self-fulfillment: Individuals with strong self-esteem are more likely to pursue activities and interests that align with their true selves. This self-fulfillment enhances life satisfaction.

6. Positive Mindset: Confidence often leads to a more positive mindset. It helps individuals focus on what's going well in their lives rather than dwelling on negativity, leading to greater satisfaction.

7. Reduced Stress: People with strong self-esteem are less likely to experience chronic stress. Lower stress levels contribute to improved overall physical and mental health, enhancing life satisfaction.

8. Personal Growth: Confidence fosters a mindset of personal growth and self-improvement. This continuous development and sense of progress contribute to a fulfilling life.

9. Happiness: Self-esteem is closely related to happiness. Confident individuals tend to experience higher levels of happiness and contentment in their daily lives.

10. Life Choices: Strong self-esteem enables individuals to make life choices that align with their values and aspirations. These choices often lead to greater life satisfaction because they are in harmony with one's authentic self.

In summary, strong self-esteem is a foundational factor for life satisfaction. It influences how individuals perceive themselves, their relationships, and their overall well-being. Cultivating and maintaining healthy self-esteem is essential for leading a more fulfilling and satisfying life.

9. EMPATHY AND COMPASSION: When you feel good about yourself, you're more likely to extend empathy and compassion to others. It promotes positive interactions and helps build a more compassionate society. Empathy and compassion are qualities often associated with individuals who possess healthy self-esteem. Here's why they are important aspects of having self-esteem:

1. Healthy Self-Image: People with strong self-esteem tend to have a positive self-image. This positive self-perception allows them to extend empathy and compassion to themselves, practicing self-care and self-compassion. When you are kind to yourself, you are more likely to extend kindness to others.

2. Greater Understanding: A positive self-image often leads to a greater understanding of one's own emotions and struggles. This self-awareness can enhance the ability to empathize with others who may be going through similar challenges.

3. Reduced Judgment: Individuals with strong self-esteem are generally less judgmental of themselves and others. They are more accepting and forgiving, which fosters empathy and compassion. When you're less critical of yourself, it becomes easier to be non-judgmental toward others.

4. Deeper Connections: Empathy and compassion are essential for building deeper and more meaningful connections with others. People with strong self-esteem are more likely to form authentic relationships based on understanding and support.

5. Conflict Resolution: Strong self-esteem often leads to better conflict resolution skills. Confident individuals can navigate conflicts with empathy and compassion, seeking resolutions that benefit all parties involved.

6. Supportive Friendships: People with healthy self-esteem tend to attract and maintain friendships with others who value and support them. These positive relationships provide opportunities to practice empathy and compassion.

7. Positive Role Models: Individuals with strong self-esteem often serve as positive role models for empathy and compassion. Their actions and behaviors inspire others to adopt similar attitudes and behaviors.

8. Contributing to a Positive Environment: Confidence and self-assurance contribute to a more positive and nurturing environment, whether at work, in the community, or at home. This fosters a culture of empathy and compassion among those around them.

9. Acts of Kindness: People with strong self-esteem are more likely to engage in acts of kindness and altruism. Their sense of self-worth enables them to extend compassion to others in need.

10. Greater Tolerance: Self-assured individuals are often more tolerant of differences and diversity. They can empathize with people from various backgrounds and perspectives, leading to greater harmony in society.

In summary, having strong self-esteem can be a catalyst for empathy and compassion. When individuals feel good about themselves, they are more likely to extend understanding, kindness, and support to others. These qualities not only benefit personal relationships but also contribute to creating a more empathetic and compassionate society.

10. POSITIVE ROLE MODELING: Individuals with strong self-esteem often serve as positive role models for others, inspiring them to develop their self-worth and confidence. Individuals with strong self-esteem often serve as positive role models in various aspects of life. Here's why this role modeling is important:

1. Inspiration: Confident individuals inspire others with their self-assuredness. Their actions and behaviors can motivate those around them to develop their own -esteem and belief in their abilities.

2. Healthy Self-Image: Positive role models with strong self-esteem demonstrate a healthy self-image. Observing their self-acceptance and self-worth can encourage others to cultivate similar feelings about themselves.

3. Assertiveness: Confident role models exhibit assertiveness and effective communication. Others may learn from their assertive behaviors, improving their unification skills and ability to express their needs.

4. Confidence Building: By witnessing confident role models, individuals may gain confidence in their abilities.

This cand to personal growth and a willingness to pursue goals with determination.

5. Mentorship: Confident individuals can serve as mentors and guides, especially in educational and professional settings. They can provide valuable guidance and support to help others reach their potential.

6. Promoting Diversity and Inclusion: Role models with strong self-esteem are often inclusive and open-minded. They can promote diversity and acceptance, fostering an inclusive environment where everyone feels valued.

7. Leadership: Confident role models often excel in leadership roles. Their leadership qualities can inspire others to take on leadership positions and contribute positively to their communities and organizations.

8. Advocacy for Self-Care: Observing individuals with strong self-esteem may encourage others to prioritize self-care, well-being, and mental health, recognizing the importance of self-compassion.

9. Positive Influence: Strong self-esteem often radiates a positive influence. People with confidence can uplift those around them, creating a more optimistic and supportive atmosphere.

10. Building a Culture of Self-Worth: Role models with strong self-esteem can contribute to building a culture where self-worth is valued and nurtured, ultimately benefiting society as a whole.

In summary, individuals with strong self-esteem have the potential to be powerful positive role models. They inspire others to cultivate confidence, resilience, healthy relationships, and a positive self-image. Through their actions and behaviors, they contribute to personal growth and the development of a more self-assured and empowered community.